CANCER HOPE:

Discovering Survivor Skills

Diane Tefft Young

ISBN 13: 9781542769402
ISBN: 154276940X

Charles Randall Lane, M.D.

"In her collection of essays, Diane gives life and meaning to the term 'cancer survivor,' by sharing her experiences and thoughtful introspection about the beauty and ugliness encountered while undergoing cancer treatment. Her perspective as a recipient of a life saving transplant followed by cancer surgery and chemotherapy is truly unique, and serves to offer hope to anyone undergoing life altering care."

Charles Randall Lane, M.D.
Cleveland Clinic
Cleveland, Ohio

FOR
ALEX AND KATIE

Table of Contents

Prologue

When I received a confirmation diagnosis of idiopathic pulmonary fibrosis at Rochester, Minnesota's Mayo Clinic in the spring of 2004, I hadn't an inkling that six years later I would receive a life-saving single lung transplant at the Cleveland Clinic.

Being diagnosed with a second life-threatening illness, stage 3C endometrial cancer in February 2015, I felt shock quickly followed by sadness. How could this be happening, again? Just one inauspicious sign (several thin ribbons of vaginal blood) that occurred three times was the single warning that my life was in potential jeopardy.

While *successfully* surviving these illnesses, I have, because of them, developed over time a resilient attitude and lifestyle. Two years post initial cancer diagnosis, I feel an emerging personal fearlessness. So unexpected! Could this be a gift from God, Mary, and the Holy Spirit? I take little credit, other than showing up and following the lead of those whom I trust.

Perhaps, you may be curious how this happened. This book's essays will provide you with windows into significant and often unexpected experiences, including developing increased resilience, that took me from feeling like, at times, a prisoner of my health diagnoses and subsequent challenges. Rather quickly, I developed a feeling of acceptance and willingness to face life as it is. Much to my surprise, as one who had lived successfully for over four years with a chronic illness, I became aware that I could *and* was living beyond my health concerns.

Friends and readers have commented, "You have strong faith." True! I am a grateful member of the Episcopal church and have benefitted from years of spiritual direction within my faith. I received stage 3C uterine cancer as a way to teach me valuable life lessons that could only be learned through this challenging experience. Many times, I have felt unaware of what the next step(s) might be. The solution was to wait and perhaps wait longer as I trusted the answer would appear at the right time. It did. Perhaps the biggest challenge I have faced has been accepting that change occurs on God's timeline, not mine!

In addition to dozens of magnificent health care professionals, I have also received support from my son, Andrew, and his two adolescent children; Alex and Katie. The most endearing memory of my grandchildren occurred six years ago, following my right lung transplant at the Cleveland Clinic. Just six days after surgery, Andrew and his family came to Cleveland for a weekend visit. As I sat up in my hospital bed to greet them, I saw Alex (age nine) and Katie (age seven) tentatively walking into my hospital room for the first time. Each had a big grin as I was handed a bouquet of brilliant autumn dahlias. Still smiling, both cautiously approached me to offer a hug. As I responded to them, I noticed and felt a gentleness and burgeoning compassion I had never witnessed before in either grandchild.

A bevy of kind and compassionate friends, my sister Melissa, and cousin Heather, have walked with me as I have laughed, cried, stumbled, and gotten back up. Their steadfast gifts of friendship and love will remain in my heart forever.

"You have always wanted to be a writer," Melissa reminded me as we were excitedly discussing my hoped-for plans for this manuscript. She was right. However, I never felt that I had a story to tell that would hold others' attention until friends suggested, following my transplant, that this rather uncommon health event with such a happy ending might be an inspirational tale that others would enjoy.

Heather, my favorite cousin, commented recently, "From the beginning, you seemed so organized about *all* of the treatment demands." I am a planner and usually try to stay up to date. There is enormous security in organization, knowing what the expectations are, and then identifying what needs to happen.

Early one warm summer Sunday morning, while sitting in the back of St. Bartholomew's Episcopal Church just before the 8:00 Rite One service began, my mind was wandering. I was recounting how fortunate I was to not only be alive, but also to be able to live a relatively normal life. Another deserving person could easily have been transplanted with the lung I received. My first book's title, *Humbled by the Gift of Life: Reflections on Receiving a Lung Transplant* was born that morning, spawned from feelings of enormous gratitude to be alive *and* to be able to be so engaged in life.

I am reminded of the often quoted 12 step recovery program slogan, "Take what you like and leave the rest." As you read *CANCER HOPE: DISCOVERING SURVIVOR SKILLS*, you may feel inspired by what you have read and perhaps at other times the opposite may be the take-away. Without question, everyone has been affected by their life experiences. This often defines how we, family members, friends, and others, respond to a cancer diagnosis. As a newly diagnosed cancer patient, I did what came naturally and what felt comfortable. I used familiar skills…ones I knew I could rely upon because I had used them so frequently for many years. It wasn't surprising that my strongest skills appeared almost effort-lessly. At other times, I had to dig deeply, very deeply, to accomplish agreed upon treatment goals. This frequently meant being willing to be open to new beliefs. I was then challenged to also develop necessary new skills as I conformed to treatment demands.

Many years ago while in the midst of divorc-ing my then-husband, I worked for several years as a career counselor. In preparation for counsel-ing others, I received training in resumé writing, interviewing, and job search strategy. "Skilling" or teaching clients how to identify their skills that they were choosing to sell to prospective employers was the backbone of our counseling strategy. While counseling others, I developed new respect and appreciation for the broad range of others' skills. It felt natural to me as I began to accept my health crisis to also create a list of skills that would aid me in getting through this challenging time as smoothly as possible.

Five years surveillance is my current treatment status. For the first two years I am scheduled to meet with my local oncologist every three months or more frequently if she, another physician, or I identify a specific need. This surveillance will be tapered to meeting twice yearly for the final three years until I reach the five year mark of being cancer-free.

The essays were written throughout the summer and fall of 2016 and winter of 2017. As you may notice, they were written independently of each other and meant to stand alone. Because of this, there is some minor repetition.

As I joined the essays together in preparation for publication, I added and updated several essays to improve the story flow for the reader. Should the reader choose to use the Thoughts for Contemplation page as a workbook page, space is allotted for writing personal thoughts and musings.

My wish is that you, the reader, will receive hope in its many faces as you read the essays, and authentically carry your message of hope as life unfolds.

1

Mimi has Cancer

Once a diagnosis of stage 3C uterine cancer was confirmed and a decision had been made about which local treatment facility would be my provider, it was time to be more open with friends, family, and grandchildren about my serious diagnosis and treatment plans.

Without question, the most challenging audience was my two early adolescent grandchildren. It was and continues to be so important to be honest with them and not frighten them at the tailend of a year of important changes within their own family. Their parents were living separately with clear plans to divorce. Although staying in the same school district, they and their many pets were moving with their mother away from the only home they had ever known and settling into a new home several miles away. Another change in their lives was a bit unwelcome.

The first week of treatment, my Patient Navigator nurse introduced herself and offered to help with questions and concerns that in a different healthcare setting might be appropriate for a medical social worker. I inquired about guidance and suggestions concerning how to tell children about having cancer and hit the jackpot. My treatment facility had age-appropriate educational cancer materials held in bright blue backpacks just waiting for Alex and Katie.

The following Sunday, as I began to tell my grandchildren about my cancer diagnosis, the intention was to use hopeful words, yet to make no promises other than I would work very hard to follow my treatment plan. Alex responded with studied silence while Katie was tearful after receiving this simple yet direct explanation of my serious cancer diagnosis.

Later that afternoon, as they left my home with their father, surprisingly they were wearing their new blue backpacks. 12 year-old Katie who was already showing signs of compassion, softly hugged me goodbye and said, "I love you, Mimi." This was an unusually caring exchange. Typically, Katie leaves my home by hugging me and saying goodbye. Several days later, I remembered generally children will accept this kind of difficult news as comfortably as it is presented to them.

Because cancer treatment is challenging for adolescents to understand especially when they aren't the patient, I shared few details about the nitty-gritty aspects of my treatment life with them. Alex and Katie spend every other weekend with their father, and it was not uncommon to see them and several friends working in my yard on hot summer weekends: cutting branches off of pine trees, trimming bushes, raking leaves, and weeding. Although, they were paid for their efforts, they always worked with good humor and fun. In early August while I was enjoying a planned treatment break after radiation and before beginning chemo infusion four, we were sitting together on the lawn during a break from their yard work. Alex looked at me and commented, "Mimi, you are as tough as nails." I don't know which adult in his life referred to me with these words, but I was amused. Resilient, yes! Tough as nails, I'm not sure. But, in Alex's eyes that day it was true. I *think* that was a compliment.

* * *

Instructions: On the final page of each essay, the reader will find three open-ended questions. These questions are designed to help the reader begin to personalize information in the essay. The reader may choose to talk with family or friends about the essay content, or possibly take notes. There is no "perfect way" or "perfect answer" as you respond to the questions below. You may also choose to skip some questions found in Thoughts for Contemplation if stopping to answer the questions interrupts the flow of reading.

THOUGHTS FOR CONTEMPLATION

1. How did you or will you tell family members about your cancer diagnosis?
2. How did you or will you share your cancer diagnosis with friends?
3. How did others respond to your honesty and vulnerability?

Space for notes and responses to
THOUGHTS FOR CONTEMPLATION

You Don't Look Sick

I attended the calling hours at St. Bart's Parish Hall of a friend's husband a few days before going to Cleveland for my hysterectomy. It was late winter, many friends were still away from the cold, windy, and snowy Midwest, enjoying warmer climates. Very close friends and immediate family were the only ones aware of my recent cancer diagnosis and pending surgery. I saw several longtime casual friends who commented at this cold February evening gathering, "You look great! How are you?" I promptly felt uncomfortable, and said, "Thank you," and avoided answering their greeting question and instead, inquired of my friends, "Did you have a nice Christmas?"

I secretly hoped we would then talk about grandchildren or their most recent visit to their Arizona home. We chatted briefly and I began to relax, thinking, "I made it through that." Not wanting to discuss *any* aspect of my life at that moment, I felt so vulnerable. Eight months later following my final chemo infusion, I saw another friend who commented as she saw me, "You look great." I recall thinking and may have said, "That is the idea." I had hoped to avoid talking about the past six months of cancer treatment. What I didn't say, but was thinking and probably is true for most of my contemporaries, cancer survivor or not, I definitely don't wake up looking this way. At 74, who does?

My transplant, in conjunction with the consequences of cancer treatment, has caused me to bruise easily. On any given day, I have at least five new or fading one-inch diameter bruises on each hand and arm. The slightest bump, it seems, creates a big red bruise which turns brown over time and eventually fades away. It is rare to see my "bare" extremities unless it's 85 degrees or above outside as my arms are usually covered by blouses, long-sleeve tee shirts, sweaters or jackets while jeans, or workout leggings hide my legs-even at the gym! Having olive skin, I always appear pale; therefore, I have a plethora of orange, peach, red, purple, green, or black clothing that I hope covers the bruises as well as adds slight color to my cheeks. I also confess to being a frequent visitor of a certain Nordstrom cosmetics counter as I attempt to keep up with changing natural make-up techniques. Three tiny tattoo dots mark the places on my abdomen used for guiding radiation techs during radiation treatment. A lengthy hysterectomy scar confirms that my body has been altered by my diagnosis and subsequent treatment. I know from transplant history, the scar will over time blend in with my skin and appear less obvious and distinctive in a year or two. The sadness and grief that I feel as my physical body has been altered is balanced by acceptance that these marks and scars are part of treatment. Do they add character to my nearly 75-year-old-body? Probably not, but they will always be a visual reminder that I *am* a survivor.

I have been prescribed a daily low dose of prednisone for over seven years. Pre-transplant, it was used to manage pulmonary fibrosis. Occasionally the dose has been increased for short periods of time and then titrated down as the infection or cause for its use has lessened. Following transplant, as a Cleveland Clinic nurse introduced eight new medications that would become lifetime meds, I learned I would continue to take five milligrams of prednisone forever. Weight gain which is frequently an issue when one takes this medication for a lengthy or even short time surprisingly has not been an issue, my weight has generally remained the same. My new dermatologist expressed surprise that my weight hasn't increased substantially because of the daily use of prednisone. My bathroom scale and a full length mirror keep my diet and weight in check.

Becoming increasingly more cautious about what I eat, I loosely follow the Mediterranean diet and no longer eat shellfish (an allergy) and frozen foods with preservatives (an allergy). I rarely eat meat and avoid pizza (calories) and casseroles (calories). Preferring fresh vegetables, fruits, and nuts while avoiding sugar, sweets, and ice cream continues to be a challenge. I often carry a water bottle, drink lots of water while I rarely drink alcohol. My affection for fresh baguettes, artisan bread, and other fresh baked goods is an addiction I wish would be removed! When eating away from home, I often query the chef, cook, or waitress to learn whether the foods are fresh and preservative-free.

I ceased visiting the gym after my second chemo infusion, I no longer had sufficient energy and the endurance to work out. For many years, I have performed a series of yoga postures and stretches at home. Despite having a healthy desire to maintain a flexible body, I didn't even have sufficient motivation to follow through with this three-times-a-week twenty-minute home routine. Sadly, for the first time in many years, during those mid-treatment four months, I didn't work out at all. The exhaustion which often accompanies treating stage 3C cancer in tandem with managing other chronic illnesses (left lung pulmonary fibrosis, a right lung transplant, cardiomyopathy, and borderline sugar diabetes) was the antecedent culprit.

Fortunately, my cancer treatment facility had a cancer wellness program. I joined this group education and workout equipment familiarization program in mid-fall. Being physically weak, my balance was off, and I had lost touch with workout safety. While getting on an elliptical machine, I fell into it. This accident caused an additional large bruise and laceration to my left leg. I avoided the elliptical machine for several months, fearing falling again because of my lack of balance. Being a cautious woman, I practiced walking on the treadmill by beginning with ten minutes and slowly increasing my time until I reached 25 minutes. I then began to alternate the treadmill with returning to the elliptical machine, increasing my time until I spent 25 minutes on the machine of choice. Today, 25 minutes on either machine is an integral part of my four times a week gym workout.

Feeling grateful that generally I don't feel or look sick, much of my energy is devoted to activities that contribute to both feeling and looking healthy. This conscious choice requires few reminders. Writing consumes a few hours each day and is a calm and gentle activity that asks for a willingness to dig deeply emotionally paired with a willingness to view life through an authentic and joyful lens. Patience and an opportunity to express my sometimes wacky sense of humor add to the pleasure I receive from seeing personal thoughts on paper.

THOUGHTS FOR CONTEMPLATION

1. Please identify additional health diagnoses.
2. Are you aware if or how these diagnoses might in the future impact your treatment?
3. How have you been affected by these diagnoses?

3

Once I had decided which local hospital oncology program would be my treatment facility, it was time to be more open with family and friends about my serious diagnosis and treatment plans.

Because of my 3C diagnosis, my oncologist recommended a "sandwich" treatment plan during which I would receive three six-hour infusions three weeks apart, followed by 28 daily radiation sessions. Treatment would end with two additional six-hour chemo infusions four weeks apart. Attempting to take all of this in, I posed a question: when will I lose my chin-length, fine, gray hair? The response was that my hair would be completely gone following the second chemo infusion. Not wanting to be stuck wearing a tired-looking, yet well-fitting OSU baseball cap all summer long and into the fall and winter, I scheduled an appointment at my treatment facility's women's cancer accessories and wig shop. Coincidentally, several years earlier, I accompanied my friend Barb, who had been diagnosed with ovarian cancer, to *her* wig selection appointment at this same shop. After speaking with Barb, she easily agreed to return the favor.

We were talking and laughing as we entered the shop that was filled with a wide selection of brightly colored hats and head coverings of all shapes, sizes, and possibilities. Because I like to be well-prepared, I had brought a picture torn from a year-old fashion magazine featuring an attractive woman with short-cropped light-blonde hair tucked behind her ears. Little did I imagine then how valuable this crumpled picture would become. The picture was offered to the wig stylist, who confidently commented; "Oh, I can do that." What a relief!

The stylist was rapidly able to see the color and style I had in mind. My olive skin was complemented by the light blonde wig I tried on, but I was encouraged to experiment with a range of different-colored and styled wigs. As I tried on a blown-out shoulder length auburn wig, the combination of my coloring and the flaming synthetic wig was beyond horrid. It was time to order the blonde wig and to leave the shop. I was told it would be available a few days after my first chemo infusion. Excellent timing.

The new wig was love and convenience wrapped together. It looked natural and real. Friends who weren't aware of my cancer diagnosis consistently commented they liked my new hair color and seemed unaware I was wearing a wig until I told them. During the next ten months, I wore my blonde wig often. It seemed to have magical powers. Although I wear minimal makeup, I would look into the mirror and see a pale, gaunt early seventies woman who looked as if she were living in a prison camp. A prisoner of my cancer diagnosis. As I looked at my reflection, my deep-set sorrowful eyes betrayed me. I began to feel the sadness about the lengthy abdominal scar created by my hysterectomy and my physical vulnerability caused by both illness and age.

Then I would put on the blonde wig and immediately feel I'd come back to life. This five-hundred-dollar wig (thanks be to God for good health insurance) had the surprising gift of enabling me to feel pretty, even attractive, at times, during this difficult year. When I wore the wig, I temporarily forgot *why* I was wearing it. The shock of being bald partially robbed me of my cultivated persona. With my blonde wig on, I felt like myself again.

Because I loved being blonde, my post-treatment plan was to have my hair stylist color my hair an almost white-blonde. Much to my surprise, as my nearly white-gray hair began to grow back, it had been affected by the harshness of chemo and came in curly; I had curls all over my head!

I did everything known to woman to encourage hair growth. I used shampoo designed to thicken thin hair and I added a maximum dose of a well-known herb that stimulates healthy nails, skin, and hair growth to my daily meds. The wig stylist offered the names of three herbs that had helped another cancer patient in her eighties grow lovely thick hair. I asked for the names and quickly drove to a local herb shop. As women in times of crisis often tend to band together, the shop herbalists consulted each other and several resource books to blend the three herbs with several carrying oils. Each night before retiring, I put three drops of the custom-blended oil into the palm of my hand and then rubbed it into my scalp. The scent was pleasant, rather musky.

What is next? I confess that as I am still not used to my curly locks, I have several summer hats from which to choose: a white fabric newly purchased wide-brimmed one and a Panama hat inherited from my well-dressed mother, Kathleen. Oh yes, the tired looking OSU baseball cap still hangs on my bedroom closet doorknob. It is saved for wearing when cutting flowers in the garden.

Best of all, I am loving this easy-going, relaxing, and at times even lazy summer free from appointments to extinguish rogue cancer cells. Recently when several women from my high school class gathered for lunch and to view a Picasso exhibit at our local art museum, I was able, on the spur of the moment, to attend. One friend, who now lives in Chicago commented, "I don't remember you having such curly hair." The response? "This is an unexpected gift from last year's chemotherapy cancer treatment." How fortunate I am to be alive, cancer-free, and sporting my newly curly hair.

THOUGHTS FOR CONTEMPLATION

1. Is chemotherapy one of your cancer treatment modalities?
2. If needed, where will you find a wig or alternative head coverings shop?
3. How do you feel about the physical changes that are happening to and may impact your body?

4

Authenticity

When I worked for over two decades as a chemical dependency counselor in hospital-based and out-patient treatment facilities, on my desk was a tiny, well-worn blue hardback book of quotations always open to the same page with the following quote from Horace:

> "It is God who can transform the
> lowest into the highest,
> who humbles the proud,
> and who causes that which is in
> darkness to become light."

I read this quote often. I felt a need to be reminded of who held the power and who was the

most magnificent change agent. For many people, this is God, a higher power or an authority
external to themselves who fulfills this role. It
is difficult to heal oneself without the support
and help of others. Holding this belief for many
years, it wasn't surprising when cancer treatment began, thoughts of this quote frequently
popped into my mind.

Quickly, I began to meet some of those others. From the telephone appointment sched-
uler to the parking lot attendant to the greeter
who smiled and acknowledged each patient who
passed over the threshold while entering the facility, these employees and staff members were
there to serve and to play a role in each patient's
treatment and hoped-for recovery.

My cancer diagnosis became real as I passed
through the revolving door entrance on my
way to the initial appointment with my oncologist. I had successfully avoided thinking about
this appointment until I handed my car keys to
the parking attendant just before entering the

facility. Unprepared and in mild shock, I felt terrified. My authentic self? Oh, yes. A volunteer who appeared at the perfect moment accompanied me to the elevator, guided me to the physician's fourth floor office waiting room, and then left as quietly as he had appeared but only after I had checked in with the receptionist. During our first appointment, I had few questions for my oncologist, I was there to observe her and to listen intently as she presented my precarious cancer diagnosis and her plans for my treatment.

I had been hospitalized at the Cleveland Clinic multiple times following transplant. Hospitals didn't scare me. What filled me with terror was the word cancer, the severity of stage 3C, *and* the awareness that I was already compromised by my lung transplant and the accompanying immunosuppressant drugs. Once again, my authentic extremely scared self.

A few months following my lung transplant surgery, I began to feel empowered. I had survived the challenging five hour transplant surgery that enabled me to breathe like everyone else as my transplanted lung worked in unison with my still very fibrotic native left lung.

Under the guidance of my spiritual director, Susannah and because I was now able to view myself as a "survivor," I soon became curious about just who my authentic self might be once my defenses were identified and were being scrubbed away. For several years, the focus of my contact with Susannah was exploring who my authentic self was. I had this opportunity to examine my life and explore which defense mechanisms I had developed over a lifetime, I was now ready, willing, and hopefully able to discard. Quite simply, these defenses were no longer useful or needed!

The authentic self tends to appear when one's persona is partially removed or discarded. As I explored, it became clearer and clearer that hanging on to no-longer-needed defenses blocked me from being that authentic self.

These defenses that had once served me well, protecting me from seeing, feeling, and believing that which I had chosen not to see, feel, and believe. It now appeared advantageous to be my authentic self.

As with most important changes, this transition to becoming more authentic required both commitment and time, but surprisingly little energy. It was hanging on to no-longer-needed defenses that was time-consuming and energy-depleting. I began to ask myself, "If I don't begin to live with fewer defenses now, when will I?"

Authenticity was about clarifying who I was and then taking steps to be that person. Further, it was about being respectful of myself and others. Being honest came naturally, but humility, vulnerability, and feeling joyful were behaviors that I saw in others and coveted mirroring. I knew life would become easier as I ridded myself of the barriers to vulnerability. I also knew that since I had used many of these defenses much of my life, they were familiar. In a pinch, sometimes without even knowing, I could and would access them in seconds.

Midway through cancer treatment, I was assigned a treatment provider who consistently seemed to be lacking in understanding *and* compassion. Having met with this person twice, it became clear, this wasn't a successful match. A request for a prompt provider change was needed. After calling my nurse and asking for a replacement provider by name, I offered to explain why the change was requested. Within several hours, I was reassigned to the requested provider. The nurse chose not to respond to my offer to explain the reason for the requested change. In the past, my habit was to make noise, too much noise, when such a request was needed and asked for. This calm, direct, and simple change in behavior left me feeling heard. As I was in the midst of exhausting radiation treatment, I had successfully wasted no energy. The bonus: I was my true self as I accomplished asking for and receiving this important staff change.

As I live more authentically, I have become aware of a greater sense of peace and calm that has begun to infuse my life. Once again, because of health issues and subsequent treatment, I had an opportunity to view myself as a survivor. This time, a cancer survivor. As I have become more self-aware, I noticed the space that had filled my heart and mind with no longer needed defenses was now open to being infused with trust and emerging fearlessness.

THOUGHTS FOR CONTEMPLATION

1. How do you describe personal authenticity?
2. Would you like to become more authentic?
3. If you decided to become more authentic, how would that change the way you interact with others?

5

A resilient lifestyle is cultivated or acquired. When I was diagnosed in the spring of 2004 with idiopathic pulmonary fibrosis, I suspect, despite taking reasonably good care of myself, no one would have identified me as being resilient. As I quickly learned about chronic illness, I also learned my diagnosis was unquestionably terminal. An Ohio Sate University pulmonologist and his student Fellow flatly informed me that I would probably live from three to five additional years. By spring 2010, it was recommended by my local pulmonologist that I should start to consider exploring a lung transplant. I was immediately open to looking into this method of extending my life. I knew I had no other realistic options. The first referral went to the Cleveland Clinic and the "back-up" referral was to be sent to an excellent transplant teaching hospital in an adjacent state. If I wanted to survive, transplantation was my single option.

Sometime during the years between diagnosis and transplant, I made a commitment to myself to do whatever it took to stay alive. And I meant it!! I was always on time for appointments with physicians, especially the Cleveland Clinic. I remember, running late for pre-transplant testing appointments because all the testing departments were running late that day. My son Andrew was trailing me and kept saying to me, "Don't worry about it, Mom" I said to him, "They are evaluating everything I do today and tomorrow. I can't mess up *anything*." At the end of my two day appointment, I was given a handout which had an additional list of seven or eight hospital-based tests that I had one month to schedule, complete, and get the results back to admissions in the Lung Transplant Department. By early August, I interviewed with the physician in charge of the lung and heart transplant department. Later in the month, I was accepted on the UNOS (United Network for Organ Sharing) lung transplant waiting list. Seven weeks later, while attending a friend's fiftieth class reunion party, I received "the call" and off he and I went to Cleveland. There was no "dry run", which frequently happens. This was the real thing. All the plans came together perfectly except getting the initial IV started. It took four sticks from three different techs before I was able to pass through the double doors on my way to surgery. Several days after surgery, one of the surgeons, as he and others were making rounds, said to me, "The stars are aligned for you."

I was discharged from the hospital after eleven days but, remained in a Cleveland area apartment hotel for another three weeks while recovering. Pre-transplant, I had developed the beginning threads of resilience skills. However, my resilience skills once I was living with my new right lung, catapulted forward as I learned how to both become protective of my transplant that I had worked so hard to receive and also to anticipate potential future health issues. Some health problems occurred without warning, others were predictable. Those who had gone before me had experienced parallel issues.

Once I arrived home, everything was set up so I could be successful. I returned to Cleveland for multiple scheduled bronchoscopies during the next two years. The "bronchs" as they are known, helped the physicians confirm all was well as my transplanted lung was integrating itself with my body. Just two months after surgery I experienced mild transplant lung rejection. I was told by my post-transplant nurse, this minor event was typical during the first year post-transplant. I decided to simply forget about the rejection. Worrying about it had no benefits, but did have the potential of making the rejection worse.

My resilience grew with each event with which I dealt. Perhaps the overriding message that finally stuck was healing and disease progression follow God's timeline, not mine. This was easy to accept as I was consistently treatment compliant. In tandem with this message was the belief that the unfolding of God's plan for my life was infinitely superior to any plan that I might create.

I learned over time to be willing to live with the ambiguity which seems to accompany illness and disease. One day I would feel healthy, happy, and have sufficient energy and enthusiasm to accomplish the plans for the day. The following day, I might feel tired and gratefully take a two hour nap. Being forewarned that this was the norm was a struggle to accept at first. It was important and necessary to be willing to let go of my illusion of control.

Letting go of control was a natural segue into trusting that my life was unfolding the way God had intended. Part of my responsibility was to get out of the way or stop interfering with God's plan. Despite all the bumps in the road, it was acceptance that became my goal.

Last, I am now learning about healthy fear-lessness. Just a bit of a challenge! All of this leads to increased resilience. I am, by nature, a cautious person. The likelihood of making a wild change that would work against my hard-earned resilience has always been low.

In the end, resilience means paying close attention to the coincidences; the unfolding of plans; listening to and remembering hopes, dreams, and wishes; being compassionate with others and myself.

THOUGHTS FOR CONTEMPLATION

1. Do you see the connection between events and resilience in your life?
2. Describe your strongest skills that contribute to your resilience.
3. What resilient skills would you like to develop in the months to come?

6

Joy

Joy in the midst of a cancer diagnosis and treatment may sound beyond next to impossible. Despite the discomfort, progressive lack of control, greater anxiety about the future, and frustration about my body's changing look and performance, and living with ongoing increased uncertainty, it was important to maintain focus and to avoid becoming sidetracked.

When I was first diagnosed, joy appeared elusive; anxiety and fear of the unknown rapidly thrust joy out of my mind. Joy had the spontaneous power of naturally elevating my mood, helping me relax, softening my feelings, and also prompted forgetting about my health circumstance. But joy was no where to be found.

Slowly, I began to recognize beautiful sunsets and to appreciate hugs and good wishes from family and friends as I got outside of myself. I looked forward to contact with grandchildren who had the magical gift of charming me and subsequently opening the door to natural and simple joy. They, in their innocent way, encouraged me to spontaneously laugh simply by spending time with them. I found myself laughing at myself for all the silly things that make me who I am. Then, I began to laugh more easily with friends about life in general. It was relaxing to forget about cancer, treatment, and the exhaustion that seemed to follow me everywhere. It took several months after treatment began to begin to see a glimmer of hope of returning to being myself. Feeling happy and like myself seemed to come and go. I was easily affected by how my treatment was progressing. Stumbling blocks (exhaustion and waiting for platelet numbers to rise) caused joy to be disappointingly intermittent.

My focus in treatment was to consistently do my best as I followed the treatment plan. This was surprisingly easy. Showing up on time *and* participating fully whether it be radiation, chemo, blood draws, or meeting with a variety of physicians was the expectation. Outside of treatment, responsibilities included eating a healthy Mediterranean diet, drinking lots of water, and getting sufficient sleep. There was a need to diligently stay on top of all other diagnoses and to follow through with previously scheduled physician and dental appointments. Because other health care providers respected the need to put cancer treatment first, they waited to make any adjustments to *their* treatment plans.

It was also my responsibility to avoid all stress. By design, my life had limited stress. Occasionally, something or someone slipped through my self-protective net. The biggest stress I experienced during this time was the frustration with slow-moving improvement in blood draw hematology test results despite following physicians' suggestions. I felt powerless. So frustrating! However, being worried about the blood draw results didn't change them, so over time deciding to let go of my self-imposed worry was the wise solution.

During mid-summer, the ability to return to hobbies which had brought me joy in the past slowly began to slip back into my life. I wrote about my treatment experience. Absent from my writing which resembled a report were feelings and the many other details that make writing come alive. My essays "read flat" as a critique peer offered in her feedback. It was the best I could do in the middle of treatment, but she was right on. Too much was happening too fast. I was incapable of catching up with my feelings. I returned to light reading. This was not only diverting, but also thought provoking at times.

I have always enjoyed yoga and working out, joining the treatment facility wellness program with its major focus on being physically active, I was grateful to be exercising again. I happily returned to the wellness program's gym and began a focused workout routine. Toward the end of treatment, I could see a glimmer of what my post-treatment life might be. Like everyone else in cancer treatment and most other health-related treatment, I could hardly wait for all the treatment to be completed.

The day before Thanksgiving, I received word that treatment had been successful; no rogue cancer cells were found in the post-treatment CT scan. I was over the moon for the next 36 hours. Sadly, on Thanksgiving night, I fell. No broken bones, fortunately, but I spent the next six months committed to and seriously involved with slowly and successfully rehabbing the damage to the right side of my body.

As a recent cancer survivor, recreating my life following treatment has offered the opportunity to both return to many of my favorite activities and also has opened space for new ways to enjoy being alive. I will always enjoy an excellent meal with good friends. I love the Episcopal Rite One service. It is perfection in its humility and direct simplicity. It is impossible to top a sunny windy day. Nothing is better than spending time with my grandchildren, Alex and Katie, whether enjoying a holiday together or a casual visit.

Over the years, I have enjoyed peak and humorous times while experiencing personal joy. Because I couldn't run any distance prior to transplant, as I approached transplant day (10.10.10), my breathing was so challenged that despite always using four liters of oxygen, walking to the end of my driveway and returning was a breathless, slow-moving struggle. I dreamed of becoming a post-transplant runner. I spoke with a member of my gym's exercise physiology staff who suggested the best way to begin to fulfill my dream was to run short sprints. After a month of sprints, I hated the stop-start aspect. I also made such a loud thumping noise as my shoes hit the track (I am not a large person) that I felt embarrassed. With relief, I gave up my fantasy sport-to-be.

In contrast, several summers ago, I took my yoga mat to the far end of the dock on one of the world's three most beautiful lakes. I enjoyed every breathtaking moment of my twenty-minute yoga routine on the dock. Quiet, simple, exquisite joy!

THOUGHTS FOR CONTEMPLATION

1. Define personal joy
2. What planned and spontaneous joyful experiences would you like to invite into your life?
3. With as much detail as possible, write about the single most joyful experience of your life.

7

Feelings

The most difficult aspect of receiving my cancer diagnosis wasn't feeling exhausted, or acting hopeful when I didn't feel that way, or knowing my "hard work" of complying with treatment expectations wouldn't guarantee being cancer-free when treatment ended. Or, even fear of dying. It was sadness and at times having to wall off my feelings so I could get through the day.

As treatment began, it was confusing distinguishing between depression and intermittent sadness as I realized and subsequently began to feel and accept the cancer diagnosis was mine... not someone else's. I felt interminably sad. Sad to my core. As I cried, it was often in conjunction with buried tears not yet shed from previous health issues. While walking into the garage before getting into my car and leaving for radiation, physician appointments, or blood draws, I would consciously put the sadness aside in order to fully engage in that morning's treatment activity.

I am needle-phobic, and the anxiety surrounding the chemo infusion needle sticks took over from sadness as the predominant emotion on chemo days. My arms' rolling veins (inherited from my mother) always have created injection difficulties. It wasn't unusual for the chemo infusion administering nurse or a tech attempting to do a blood draw to need to do a second or even third stick to accomplish the task. I was used to this. Much to everyone's consternation, in the last six years during five hospitalizations, I have also effortlessly blown a rather large number of IVs.

Fortunately, my sadness wasn't depression. Sadness is a predictable and normal response to a serious health diagnosis or prognosis as well as to other expected or perhaps unexpected life disappointments or challenges. When sadness was put aside, I was able to thoroughly enjoy my life as other more typical feelings emerged. I sought opportunities to spend time chatting with good friends. Spending time with my grandchildren as they worked in my yard was a welcome, relaxing, and happy diversion. Both Alex and Katie have an enviable, spontaneous adolescent sense of humor. They helped keep sadness at bay.

While I longed to visit my gym, initially, I didn't have the energy or stamina to enjoy being there. Unfortunately, I also felt clumsy and awkward at times because of not working out. Being one who relishes shopping for new clothes, I avoided shopping, fearing if I bought new clothes, I might not live long enough to wear and enjoy them. Yes, death and dying were on my mind, flickering in and out of my thoughts when I wasn't busy. I quite successfully stayed busy most of the time. Thanks be to God, days passed when these thoughts never entered my mind.

About five years ago, once my relationship with spiritual director Susannah was well established, she regularly began to introduce the topic of compassion. My history of working for many years as a counselor made it easy to feel compassion for others. The true challenge was to feel compassion for myself. Initially feeling this emotion for myself felt awkward. However, in the last few years, there have been multiple opportunities to practice this grown-up valuable skill.

Multiple illnesses have crossed my path, including the disease which created the need for a lung transplant. Several years later, I contracted difficult-to-diagnose Nocardia pneumonia. I discussed this serious diagnosis with my post-transplant nurse, John. Hoping to speak with another transplant patient who also had been diagnosed with this type of pneumonia, I asked him about the possibility of talking with another survivor, a Nocardia pneumonia survivor. John glanced away and then looked down. I looked directly at him and said, "They are all dead, aren't they?" He nodded. There was some thought that pneumonia may have been acquired from bacteria found in garden dirt, but this was never confirmed. Nonetheless, I promptly ceased all gardening.

The following fall, during Columbus Day weekend, I ate a packaged frozen Chinese dinner which caused an immediate allergic reaction. After several hours of endless itching and scratching, I called the Cleveland Clinic Lung Transplant on-call physician. After asking multiple questions, this physician said decisively, "Call 911, now." I waited outside my home in the cool night air for the paramedics to arrive. Once inside their van, an IV was started just before I ceased breathing. I was taken to a local hospital's ICU. The plan was for me to be life-flighted to the Cleveland Clinic. However, four days of consistent foggy and rainy Ohio October weather delayed my flight to Cleveland. While waiting, I remained in the local hospital's ICU. I have no memory of the forever lost four days. After being life-flighted to the Cleveland Clinic, I awoke angrily fighting the ICU staff as they attempted to extubate me. Once the breathing tube was removed, I was transferred from the ICU to the familiar lung transplant floor.

That was the last straw. My unrelenting determination about *not* being re-hospitalized emerged. Quickly, I became cautious about everything I ate and began to wash my hands frequently. While mandatory allergy testing indicated no identifiable allergies, my local allergist suggested that an unknown food preservative was the probable culprit. I began eating fresh food almost exclusively. When eating in restaurants, I query the chef or waiter to confirm that the meal is entirely fresh— free from all preservatives. A recent shellfish allergy has appeared. The probable cause of this allergy is that my lung transplant donor also may have experienced this same allergy. Despite several failed attempts to learn the identity of my transplant donor, I remain respectfully in the dark. I am exceedingly grateful to her and her family.

Becoming more self-protective has been my response to life's mounting physical anomalies. While I have the beginning threads of self-compassion because of my multiple health-related diagnoses and crises, thus far I have experienced very little physical pain. Is this because of a high pain threshold? Perhaps. I am reminded once again, that God is in charge of teaching me valuable lessons about life including reminding me how grateful I am to both be alive and to be able to be so engaged in my ever-evolving life.

THOUGHTS FOR CONTEMPLATION

1. What feelings did you have about cancer before being diagnosed with cancer?

2. What are predominant feelings that you have felt after being diagnosed with cancer?

3. Have friends or family members shared their feelings of concern for you with you?

8

Life's Challenging Moments

When my chronic lung disease diagnosis was confirmed at the Mayo Clinic in 2004, it was difficult for friends and family to know how to react. This was understandable. Neither did I. How does one learn to "be sick?" I knew no one with a chronic illness. Neither of my parents could claim such a medical history. My maternal grandfather, forced to give up his dental practice because of progressive multiple sclerosis, was bedridden when I was a young child. He died before I entered first grade. If his wife, my grandmother were living today, she probably would be diagnosed as having experienced a stroke. My mother although active early in her life, after age 55, experienced a series of health issues that required multiple surgeries and also a diagnosis of cardiomyopathy. Both of my father's parents successfully survived late-life cancer. My grandfather died of heart disease while, my grandmother, died in her late eight-ies from old age. My father, although suffer-ing through stress-related short-term physical challenges, was healthy enough to play eighteen holes of golf at age ninety-five a few days before his unexpected death from a stroke.

Without role models for how to be sick, I hadn't a clue about what to do after receiving my diagnosis of idiopathic pulmonary fibrosis, also known as IPF. It was suggested by my Mayo Clinic diagnostic pulmonologist that once re-turning home, I should enroll in a two-month, out-patient pulmonary rehab program. I learned valuable lessons while in rehab: when to wear a face mask, how to avoid contagious sick people, and how weather and climate affected my breath-ing. To my astonishment, it was apparent that

I was not as sick as ninety percent of the other group members. Rehab gave my disease, despite its life threatening reality, a context in which I could view myself in relationship to others with the same or similar pulmonary diagnoses.

Following rehab, as instructed, I returned to working out and participating in mat Pilates and yoga classes at my gym. As expected, my disease progressed, but relatively slowly in the beginning. I found an excellent local pulmonologist, a high school classmate of my younger sister, Melissa. Because I didn't want to think or hear about the predictable end result of my disease (death), I wandered away from this pulmonologist. He, of course, was wiser than I and when I didn't return for appointments for over a year, he kindly but firmly helped me understand that I needed to meet with him every six months. I have never been a particularly avoidant person; however, the thoughts of death and dying brought on by idiopathic pulmonary fibrosis successfully drove me from keeping appointments with him.

Disease progression (increased stiffening of both lungs because of lung scarring) became a growing concern as it was becoming more difficult to simply breathe. This physician was the first person to discuss lung transplantation with me and he subsequently made the referral to the Cleveland Clinic lung transplant program. His referral saved my life.

I have been extremely fortunate to have kind and supportive friends. I have made a concerted effort to refrain from developing or holding on to friendships that appear even mildly disrespectful and thoughtless. However, a few people have slipped through my self-protective net. I am rarely confrontational even when someone is disrespectful or thoughtless. My anticipated follow-up is to have no planned future contact with the disrespectful person.

Whenever I have thought about why I have ceased contact with someone, I have noticed, a common thread, the disrespectful person lacks compassion. I have observed that they may have experienced histories of serious health issues within their families, but they themselves aren't chronically ill. These health issues might have changed their family dynamics. A spouse or a child may be or have been chronically ill or may have died. In the situations I have experienced, the disrespectful person appears to be unaware of their own lack of recovery from the pain brought on by the important loss that has occurred in their lives. Their pain, disguised as disrespect, is tossed onto unsuspecting and inappropriate persons.

I tend not to confront others for several reasons. When people are disrespectful or unkind it is almost always about *their* behavior and generally has little to do with the target of their hapless feelings. Since people don't usually strike out, unless they are emotionally hurting, I ask myself; "Do they have a significant unhealed wound?" Probably yes, but they may be completely blind to it. By striking back, life is given to *their* disrespect and often encourages their lack of compassion and their blindness to come out even more. Recently, when someone was over-the-top disrespectful, I woke up in the middle of the night praying for the person. This was a nod or reminder to pray for this person at least once a day. Praying is known to often soften the attitude toward the one in pain and also often may be an invitation to open the door for forgiveness.

I have occasionally had contact with people who voiced thoughts of "poor you" directed toward me. Since I am unclear why they have this attitude, it appears this comment has little to do with me and again, I suspect, everything to do with them. Apparently, they haven't a clue about how grateful I feel to be alive and to be able to be so engaged in life. Being close to death more than once has offered a new perspective about and appreciation for life.

The other behavior that I find to be unknowing occurs when someone thinks they know just how someone else must feel in relationship to their health and the experiences it has brought into their life. I have had naive people assume or infer I am angry, when I am accepting of this situation. Since we all have completely different life experiences, how could another person honestly know how someone else is feeling? I appreciate people who inquire about how I feel about my health circumstance. In some odd way, people who don't inquire may incorrectly assume that everyone feels just as they do. These people tend to project their feelings, what-ever they are, onto unsuspecting others. After I have become aware of their habit of projection, I tend to steer clear of them.

I am grateful to a host of kind, caring, and supportive friends. Close family members also have been present when needed. Fortunately, somehow just the right friend seems to show up at the perfect time. The kindness and compassion that has filled my life continues teaching me over time how to be a compassionate friend who hopefully appears with a spontaneous delicious sense of humor!

THOUGHTS FOR CONTEMPLATION

1. What kinds of unexpected behavior have "friends" displayed?
2. How did you respond to their behavior?
3. How do you like and expect to be treated at this time in your life?

9

Spirituality

Priest Albert played a valuable role in leading me to my spiritual director, Susannah. We met in his spacious and cosy office one dreary, wet, late-winter afternoon eight years ago, just months after he had accepted the call as priest-in-charge of St. Bartholomew's Episcopal Church. I *thought* the purpose of our meeting was to become acquainted. As we talked, I spontaneously talked about, until that moment, my unspoken wish to find a spiritual director. Albert suggested several Diocese of Southern Ohio educational and training organizations that might know who was available within the diocese to provide the requested service. During the next two weeks, disappointing dead-end phone calls produced no viable candidates. Then, out of the blue, Susannah's name was recommended. Her name sounded familiar, we were members of the same local affiliate of a respected national women's volunteer and leadership training organization, yet we had never met.

During our initial phone contact, Susannah shared she and her husband were in South Florida and planned to return to their Ohio home in late spring. Several months passed before our first appointment. The process of spiritual direction began as we introduced ourselves and I expressed my developing hopes about the direction of our future meetings. Admittedly, I was in the dark about how life changing as well as affirming this mystical and mysterious sharing process would become. Little did I know, I had found a spiritual companion who would fulfill a multitude of roles evolving as needed. Susannah's guidance has been experienced as: a wise older sister, a caring mother, and a friend with whom I could laugh uproariously about my foibles, short-comings, and joys. But, equally important, I could speak with her about deep feelings of sadness and grief brought on by mounting life-threatening health concerns. As I learned to trust Susannah, I further benefitted from her vast knowledge about family systems especially related to the multiple roles I have played: daughter (until May 2013 when my father died), mother, grandmother, sister, cousin, compassionate and fun-loving friend, and at times go-to person for those with unanswered chemical dependency concerns.

Much to my surprise, over the years, I have learned that we grew up in rather similar suburban families, are the oldest child in our families of origin, have Master's degrees in the counseling field, and have upon occasion assumed leadership roles within the broader community. Surprisingly, we both have a fascination with the beauty of color and an affinity with Mary, the mother of Jesus. Because of the necessity for clear and expected boundaries, we may have shared other life experiences however, I am simply unaware of them.

It was Susannah with whom I wept and wept from a place deep in my soul just days before

going to transplant. I never wavered from believing that I would receive a healthy lung for
transplant in time. However, I was so focused on
staying alive, I hadn't considered what life would
be like post-transplant, or how impaired this
major surgery might leave me. Or, what would
happen if my body rejected my new lung and
left me with a single poorly functioning native
left lung? I had no answers, I hadn't the courage
nor bravery to ask and to think that far ahead. I
knew one thing, I would rapidly succumb without a lung transplant.

As with all lung transplant patients, my
breathing deteriorated quickly as I inched closer to death. I was so sick, when I met with the
physician-director of the transplant program
just days before transplant, she told me when
life became too physically challenging, I could
call her, and she would request that a hospital
small jet be summoned to Central Ohio to pick
me up and transport me to the Cleveland Clinic.
My life would then be sustained on the hospital
transplant floor until a perfect match lung was

found. How reassuring this was to hear. It was only later that I was able to see my denial and then began to accept how close to death I actually was. Historically, pulmonary fibrosis (my lung disease) progresses rapidly toward the end of life.

Having been a counselor in the field of addiction for many years as well as having regularly attended Al-Anon meetings for over a decade, I felt I had a solid grasp and understanding of powerlessness. Once diagnosed with stage 3C cancer, this belief was challenged. I had then and continue to have a deficit in my ability to develop a healthy blood supply. My body's ability to snap back after five chemotherapy infusions and 28 daily radiation sessions and grow healthy blood cells progressed slowly. A partial solution during cancer treatment was an infusion of two units of A negative blood. This occurred twice. To date, additional progress has been made, but during a recent appointment with my hematology oncologist, I inquired about what I might do to assist with or speed up this process. He shared there was nothing beyond what I had been doing for the last nine months…eating a healthy diet, participating in daily physical exercise, avoiding all stressful situations, and enjoying my life. The antecedent of my blood manufacturing difficulties is the required transplant immunosuppressant drugs that accompany all transplants.

Several years ago, I became aware that Susannah kept bringing me back to the topic of compassion. Compassion for others seemed to be easier to feel than compassion for myself. Toward the end of my years working as a chemical dependency counselor, I began to feel a greater grasp of the compulsion which accompanies addiction. Compassion developed readily for those who demonstrated self-responsibility. Once I had integrated those feelings, I was naturally lead to feelings of compassion for all who suffer. With a history of being "hard on myself" it has taken time, perseverance, and patience to become more self-compassionate.

Limited energy determines how active I am able to be each day. The slow but steady progress that I have made after a no-broken-bones but serious fall (tripping over a curb in the dark and landing fortunately in soft grass) on Thanksgiving night last year has been a challenge. Six weeks of physical therapy in tandem with weekly massage and acupuncture began my rehabilitation. Despite working out at my gym three times a week coupled with twenty minutes of home stretching on the three alternate days lead to slow and uneven progress. After four to five months of being frustrated and annoyed because physical therapists and massage therapists were unable to project how well or even if my seventy-four year old body would bounce back and repair itself, I decided that an incentive might speed up the progress. Continuing with my home and gym workouts, the planned reward when I was close to being back to normal was either a weekly yoga class or a Pilates-on-the-Reformer class. These classes were designed to maintain or improve my physical stamina and agility. I am almost ready to explore the classes thanks to consistent hard work at the gym and wise counsel, acupuncture, and cupping from my sports medicine physician.

Perhaps the biggest difference in the last two years is an increasing awareness of simply accepting my physical limitations. When *my* plans aren't being adhered to, I am more accepting and aware that there is perhaps a better plan. When I become tired, I have become more accepting and subsequently more selective about how time is being spent. I remain somewhat intolerant of wasting my available time because time and energy have become so precious. As time has passed, I have developed a greater awareness of how to make the most of my available energy. I recently eliminated several monthly commitments simply to see if life would be simpler without these activities. Or perhaps, I would prefer to be occasionally involved. While my commitment to myself to write this book has significantly impinged upon the rest of my life, I feel grateful that I made the decision to write this book this year. It is not surprising, that writing this collection of essays has been a rewarding aspect of my healing. Once again, I am intrigued by how exquisitely all of life's puzzle pieces fit together.

THOUGHTS FOR CONTEMPLATION

1. What is compassion?
2. How do you feel when others treat you with compassion?
3. How do you demonstrate compassion for yourself? For others?

10

Trust to Fearlessness

Being diagnosed with endometrial cancer in early 2015 remains my single most frightening life experience. Just one inauspicious sign (several tiny thin ribbons of vaginal blood) that occurred three times, was the only warning that all was not well and my life was in potential jeopardy.

As an exploration of the source of the warning sign began, I always asked for and fortunately received first-available physician appointments. Three months passed as I progressed from an initial appointment with my primary care physician to a local gynecologist who completed a uterus exploration and minor scraping to a local gynecological surgeon who, following a D and C (dilation and curettage), informed me of my stage 1 endometrial cancer diagnosis.

Last, I had a consult with a Cleveland Clinic gynecological oncology surgeon. Because of my history with the Cleveland Clinic, I agreed to return to the same hospital for the next step, a hysterectomy. The surgery was complicated by unexpected adhesions and an accidental bowel nick that demanded on-the-spot repair.

What a surprise to learn after the four-hour surgery that my diagnosis wasn't stage 1 cancer as originally thought, but stage 3C. Cancer had spread to four neighboring lymph nodes. Clearly, the diagnosis was more serious than I had initially been told.

Treatment success was challenged by my permanently compromised immune system. Using my laptop computer, I confirmed during an online search that my five-year chance of cancer survival was slightly less than fifty percent. There appeared to be no way to factor in the survival odds complicated by my nearly five-year-old lung transplant.

Life felt as if it were spinning out of control. What I did know was that I would faithfully follow my local cancer hospital's treatment plan (chemotherapy and radiation) spread over six months *and* I would hold a positive attitude despite what was occurring to and around me.

I applied an Al Anon slogan, "Act as if" to my life while in treatment. I acted as if treatment was working. I focused on what was happening that day, and only occasionally referred to what had happened in the past or would happen in the future. When I stayed in the present moment there wasn't time nor space for fear or anxiety. I am a cautious person already; fear and anxiety offered no benefit. None.

Over time, I became tired of being a patient, tired of *all* the additional blood draws and angry about having to put treatment ahead of everything else in my life. I knew it was "normal" to feel this way.

It felt as though an invader had moved in and had taken over my life. I didn't want my "old life" back, because I was being changed by the experience. I simply wanted a life not driven by medical care.

I promised myself I would identify and try to eliminate *all* stressful people, places, and things as quickly as they were identified. Easier said than done, but there was no question in my mind, I would do my very best. But, would that be enough? Being able to count on myself was a given, and whether I liked it or not, cancer treatment had to be the centerpiece of my life from Easter, 2015 until Thanksgiving, 2015.

Reflecting on 2015, it seems miraculous that I was able to walk through this difficult time somewhat gracefully due in part to the skilled professionals at both my local cancer treatment facility and the Cleveland Clinic. As my cancer facility took the lead, they were supported and educated about the effects of my transplant and accompanying meds on my cancer treatment by the experts of Cleveland Clinic's lung transplant program. Further support was felt from immediate family members (son Andrew and his adolescent children), close friends, and friends who simply popped up at just the right moment.

A variety of friends volunteered to transport me to and from the five chemotherapy infusions. Despite all the blood draws and injections during the last six years, I still don't like needles. I consistently felt anxious about this aspect of treatment. I live just ten minutes from my cancer facility. With careful planning, always a calm and soothing friend arrived at my home to take me to my early morning six hour infusion. One friend was curious about the process. She accepted the invitation to join me in my infusion room for the initial ninety minute chemo set-up. When it came time to retrieve me six hours later, she had temporarily lost her keys!

Another friend responded to a different plea for help. A week after I returned home from my Cleveland hysterectomy, I couldn't stop throwing up. I called a friend to get a second opinion about whether I should call 9-1-1. Upon arriving at my home and taking one look at me, she quickly concurred, call 9-1-1 *now*. I spent another weekend in the hospital, this time entering the hospital where I would soon receive cancer treatment.

During the radiation treatment filled summer, a longtime friend appeared who not only is an expert gardener herself, but also has ready access to the crew who cares for her gardening needs. Together they designed and installed an entirely new expanded front garden. Now, on either side of the front walk from the driveway to the front door, the garden is filled with myrtle, various varieties of day lilies, grape hyacinths, coneflowers, daffodils, iris, Russian sage, lavender, Japanese wisteria, and many other colorful perennial flowers. Three large landscape rocks as well as a large blown glass and metal sculpture in the shape of a spider greet those who approach the front door.

Additionally, a variety of friends graciously treated me to lunch or dinner and accepted me for being where I was…frightened by my serious diagnosis and at the beginning of the not-yet-traveled winding road of treatment. I felt touched and humbled by their understanding and compassion.

I was also aware of the presence of my spiritual director Susannah as well as my belief in the protectiveness of God, Mary, and the Holy Spirit. I trusted that friends and the ever-present spiritual figures were active in my life for a reason! Unquestionably, I needed and benefited from their kindness as well as their enduring ability to laugh with me at the unexpected timely and funny happenings that occurred.

In retrospect, I accepted my health scare and never asked "why me" because I sensed that developing cancer and participating fully in the necessary treatment was happening to teach me valuable lessons I could learn *only* through this experience. Trust in myself continued to develop along the way and substantially aided me in letting go of the fear that almost always accompanies serious illness. Without question, I value my life, relationships with family and friends, and time on earth in a way I never ever could have before. Once again, it is with overwhelming gratitude that my life is *now* enhanced with a developing healthy fearlessness.

THOUGHTS FOR CONTEMPLATION

1. Please describe trust. Please describe fear-lessness.
2. Identify significant experiences in your life when you have felt trust.
3. Identify significant experiences in your life when you have felt fearless.

11

Becoming Fearless

The first time I heard fearless in conjunction with my name, I was enjoying a late-lunch rare roast beef sandwich with a distant cousin-friend at our gym's restaurant. This happened almost six years post-transplant and nine months after being designated a cancer survivor by my treatment facility.

I was in the midst of learning how to balance the energy tempo of my life. An active hour in the gym was easily doable yet social situations of any sort were far more energy demanding and energy depleting. It was easier to schedule one activity each day, rather than commingling multiple activities that consistently produced the beginning threads of exhaustion. It became clear that not having sufficient energy undermined my hoped-for active daily schedule.

Predictably, there were several major projects which were the foci of my life: writing this manuscript of cancer-themed essays as well as initiating a health manuscript reviewer search. I was also reviewing new car options as the lease on my current car was ending in several months. I was caring for my home (not the yard and garden), enjoying meeting friends for lunch or dinner. I also attempted to simplify my life by selling and donating unneeded clothing, furniture, jewelry, and books, in addition to an odd assortment of inherited family "stuff." All in an effort to streamline and simplify my day-to-day life into becoming more authentic and joyful. No stress allowed.

When thinking about fearlessness, I asked myself, "How have I learned to live without fear?" This major jump in managing my life has occurred incrementally over the past twelve years. However, the greatest progress has happened during the last six years. Learning how to live comfortably with a single-lung transplant has been the foundation or platform for learning how to live less fearfully. This gradual shift has required a new openness and a willingness to request help when needed. During this time, I have asked countless people (some known and others unknown) for help.

There is a certain humility that needs to be present when asking the world for help. Earlier in life, I simply didn't have the humility to ask for help. Humility was foreign to me. I didn't feel comfortable being that vulnerable. I didn't grow up surrounded by this valuable quality. Neither of my parents was comfortable being humble. Vulnerability is an additional aspect of asking for help. Always, my internal question has been, "What will I do if the person I have asked for help says no?" The obvious answer is to ask another qualified person to help. But once turned down, it isn't always easy to become courageous, more vulnerable, and ask again. However, it is no surprise, often when someone is unable to help, the second or third choice may be the better or best choice.

Receiving a stage 3C cancer diagnosis, put me in an exceptionally vulnerable spot. I knew from diagnosis forward, the survival odds were stacked against me. This fact in addition to consistently feeling a progressive degree of fatigue and intermittent sadness left me feeling that I needed to develop humility quickly. As a woman, it is an exceptionally leveling experience to be robbed of all your hair and then be placed in a room of others with a cancer diagnosis who are humbled as they too may be receiving chemo and or radiation. Despite the enormous benefits of these treatment techniques, there is a lengthy list of potential side effects. Looking into a mirror and seeing my familiar facial features but no hair always left me feeling beyond sad.

Having grown up in a family where the four children were unaware of the somewhat hidden or unacknowledged pervading attitude of entitlement was my experience. This was the manner in which our parents moved through life. As I entered cancer treatment, it became clear it was time to let go of any shreds of this core belief and behavior. It was humility that I was seeking in the months and years ahead.

The humility that I longed for in an odd way was complemented by my early decision to be exceptionally polite with *every* treatment provider with whom I had contact whether it be the gentleman who parked my car, the man who drew my blood; and the varied nurses who assisted with physician's orders in chemo, patient navigation, in the physician's office, and the multiple physicians themselves. I was the first transplant patient my oncologist had ever treated. Because my required transplant meds impacted my blood draw results, I asked my post-transplant nurse to educate my oncology nurse about the short and long term effects of my transplant and required meds had on my overall health, cancer treatment, and blood draw results.

Having seen the disappointing results from years of counseling addiction patients who chose not to be treatment compliant, I was determined to be treatment complaint. I allowed myself no wiggle room. None.

As sad as I felt when treatment began, I knew that both my treatment path as well as the outcome were in God's hands. I never wavered from this core belief. With this certainty firmly in place, there was no role, no space for fear. It became clear to me early on, that a firm belief in God had the power to shove fear aside. As fear was edged out of my life, it lost power, control, and influence in my daily life. This kept the space open for me to see and to feel more clearly that God was indeed in charge. How many times and in how many ways did I need to be reminded?

I did not want to die. I felt then and I feel now there are still many things I want to accomplish. It is in God's hands when and how I will depart this earth. This belief was and continues to be an enormous relief. Fear takes a huge amount of energy to sustain. I didn't want to waste any precious resources on unhealthy and disempowering fear.

As feeling fearless is rather new to me, I am curious how this will continue to impact the many facets of my life. I welcome this transition. I have already noticed one change, I am becoming less affected by people who lack civility. There is no space for this attitude in my life and I quickly remove myself from these energy-depleting people and situations. This change opens space for the respectful, kind, and creative people and experiences that I welcome.

THOUGHTS FOR CONTEMPLATION

1. What does it mean to "live fearlessly"?
2. What does it mean to "live with humility?"
3. Are you able to ask for help when needed?

12

Survivor's Gift

As word spread about my diagnosis, I heard from a friend that Gillian (a sculptor and ceramist who I have known for many years) had also been diagnosed several years earlier with stage 3C endometrial cancer. My friend gave me Gillian's phone number and encouraged me to call. When I reached Gillian several days later, she shared she had received treatment at a local cancer-designated hospital. Quarterly PET (positron emission tomography) scans have confirmed that she remains cancer-free. This news infused me with hope in a way no other good news possibly could. Gillian encouraged me to call her any time if I had questions or simply wanted to talk. This was a welcome and most appreciated offer—and one I eagerly accepted.

During the ensuing months of treatment, she and I remained in contact. Gillian who is a bit of a free spirit has a delicious sense of humor. If anyone had overheard us chatting and laughing on the phone, more often than not, they might have been amazed, even shocked, at the source of our humor.

The Wednesday morning before Thanksgiving, 2015, I was scheduled for a CT (computed tomography) scan to determine if treatment had been successful. As time inched closer to this scan, anxiety took over. I became increasingly anxious-so anxious, I was no longer hungry. Nothing, not even festive holiday meals sounded appealing. The appointment was scheduled for 8:00. Several hours later, as I was driving home, my cell phone rang. My oncology nurse was the first to tell me that no cancer had been found in the scanned area. The following Monday, I met with my oncologist, who referred to me as a "survivor." The term survivor has never held much significance for me. However, in that moment, I felt for an instant like a sparkly star high in the night sky. In partnership with my treatment facilities various providers, supportive friends and family, and under God's governance umbrella, I had indeed become a cancer survivor.

I was just becoming used to my survivor status when I was awakened one night by a text announcing a long ago neighbor's current dangerous and startling health diagnoses. Rereading the text, I learned that Lainie had experienced a heart attack in late October. She was further diagnosed with lung cancer. Several weeks after Christmas, Lainie had surgery in which a portion of her right lung was removed. Sadly, she also learned at that time that her cancer had spread to five neighboring lymph nodes. Her body wasn't yet strong enough for the harshness of cancer treatment. I awoke the next morning and reread my phone message. Former neighbors responded to Lainie's health crisis by wanting to send her flowers and cards, to pray for her, and to connect her with an excellent cardiologist-relative. As I thought about how I might be of service to Lainie, tears began to fill my eyes as I realized how similar our health histories were. I quickly became aware that the best thing I could do for Lainie was to be myself, offering her the authentic gift of hope, laughter, and compassion just as my mentor-friend Gillian had given me.

THOUGHTS FOR CONTEMPLATION

1. Would you like to be paired with a cancer mentor?
2. What qualities do you seek in the ideal mentor?
3. If you decided you could benefit from a cancer mentor, how would you find one?

13

Life: One Year Post-Treatment

Despite a rather gloomy picture, the weather today is a reminder that winter is coming. It is chilly, windy, and peppered with intermittent rain showers. The sun has been hidden all day. Hoping to feel comfortable on this first autumn chill-to-the-bone day, I am sitting in my office just off the living room listening to the beautiful sounding trumpet of Chris Botti and feeling ever so happy and grateful to be alive. It is almost one year since October, 15, 2015, my final six hour chemo infusion day. I remember the date so clearly, almost five years and five days since my right lung transplant. I have just completed an intensive new car search. I visited five dealerships and as it is almost the last day of September, car bargains abound. This is not only the end of the month but also the end of the 2016 new car sales year. I have narrowed my choices to two different Japanese made cars, each offering specific advantages. The decision is almost made, I am waiting for the answers to two final questions from one dealership and then tomorrow the choice will be shared with the sales people with whom I have been speaking. I have always loved cars, however, this has been an exhaustive and exhausting process.

Last year is now a memory. I *never* imagined that one year later I could and would be as active as I am and also feel a surprising sense of peace and acceptance about my life. As much as I dislike the term "new normal," life has a freshly-established flexible yet steady rhythm. Taking excellent care of my health is the logical and natural centerpiece. Writing and the day-to-day promotional activities attached to this work… yes, even this early in the process; spending time and often enjoying a meal with friends; participating in almost daily physical exercise; reading; and caring for my home, these activities fill my days. Life feels full of experiences that are meaningful and valued. I have reluctantly begun to accept that I will always be challenged by having sufficient energy to accomplish everything I would like to do each day. I am reminded to move slowly and keep my focus on the activity in which I am involved. This single thought helps to avoid feeling overwhelmed or exhausted. As I plan each day, I remember to schedule sufficient breaks so I am able to fully engage in life. This is easily accomplished. Because social occasions are both fun and energy-demanding, I rarely schedule two such occasions back-to-back or even on the same day. An entire year has been required to develop this rhythm and balance. It is an ongoing and evolving process.

Several days ago, I met with a new physician, a nephrologist. After examining the results of four separate summer blood draws and interviewing me, she determined that a change in medication was necessary. Amazing but true; one medication was changed from daily use to take-as-needed and one cardiac med's dose was cut in half. I now take the medication in the morning; the evening dose has been eliminated. I will visit with my Cleveland Clinic cardiologist in a month. What will he say about this change, which is designed to eliminate low blood pressure?

The result from calculating how much time is spent each month on my health was a big surprise. Between ordering and picking up meds, filling the med boxes each week, I spend at least three hours each month staying on top of them. Scheduling and attending physician and dental appointments averages another eight hours, participating in at least one blood draw adds an additional hour, reviewing all insurance and Medicare claims including frequent follow-up phone calls and filing the paperwork is three more hours.

Because working out at my gym and at home requires another eight hours each week or 35 hours monthly, I spend a minimum of 50 hours each month staying on top of my physical health. These numbers are based upon a typical month without health or other emergencies. A minimum of two days each year is devoted to traveling from my Central Ohio home to the Cleveland Clinic for check-ups with my lung transplant program nurse-coordinator, pulmonologist, and cardiologist. I usually travel to Cleveland with my son as it gives us an opportunity to catch up. Andrew works out-of-town all week as a project manager for a global company. In addition to enjoying spending time with him, should there be a major health change, he is available to hear physician updates, to ask questions, and for support. This system has been amended by circumstance and need many times, but in general, it has worked extremely well.

My two grandchildren live in an adjacent county one-half hour away. As adolescents, they spend most of their time involved with school and sports activities and their friends. Sadly, I see them less frequently than I used to, and naturally miss seeing them. While they live with their mother, they spend every other weekend with their father who lives nearby. Time is especially precious in their young lives. Alex will be driving in April and before he realizes it, he will be in college studying engineering. Katie who is a bit of a free spir-it and a definite animal-lover has aspirations of becoming a veterinarian while also having a strong affinity for the arts (photography). There is nothing I enjoy more than spending time with my two favorite people and hearing their take on the changing world in which we live. I have offered to hold Thanksgiving din-ner at my home this year for Andrew and his children, his significant other, her two adoles-cents, and her mother. What a privilege to feel well enough to plan, organize, and jointly cook one of my favorite holiday meals. When I have successfully persuaded Andrew to find and to return my turkey roaster pan, I'll be ready to move forward.

How grateful I feel to have trusted friends with whom I feel comfortable. They have walked with me during difficult times, gently supported me through moments of sadness during treatment, and celebrated with me last fall when I reached the five-year mark as a lung transplant recipient. One friend with the same diagnosis who has been in successful post-cancer treatment surveillance for several years, gently mentored me as I progressed through the different treatment modalities as well as the stages of grief. Gillian was a beacon of hope when I needed to "see" hope. I was simply terrified of the potential outcome of treatment, fearing because of my serious stage 3C diagnosis complicated by my encumbering transplant immunosuppressant meds I might not survive. When I became fearful, I would think about Gillian, her three years of survivor status, and my fear would gradually dissipate. Then, I would return to being able to stay in the present moment. It would have been a lonely, lonely ride without family and dear friends.

Fortunately, I have always enjoyed being physically active. Once I was in the final stage of treatment, I joined my hospital's cancer wellness program. Program staff members mapped out a personalized re-entry workout routine and provided dietary education. Amended several times, the initial wellness program plan remains the backbone of my workout. Now, over a year later after my Thanksgiving night fall, the only noticeable effect from the fall is a slight limp that appears when I am tired. Currently exercising at eight separate stations as well as walking on the treadmill or using an elliptical machine for twenty minutes four days a week, my exercise routine is predictably effective. This is combined with, on alternate days, two twenty minute home yoga stretching sessions each week.

Most people who write are naturally frequent readers. I fall into this category and tend to read best sellers, often exchanged with friends. Although not a member of a book club, I look forward to becoming a member of such a group in the near future. Recently, a friend from a former writer critique group expressed interest in establishing a new critique group. Our initial planning meeting is scheduled for later this month.

Although currently I don't have assistance with the cleaning and minor maintenance of my home, I am responsible for its internal and external upkeep and maintenance. I could easily hand off many of these duties. My son and grandson are available for moving furniture, hanging paintings, replacing outdoor concrete steps, and sometimes cleaning gutters. A big help! I try to stay on top of major maintenance issues e.g. changing furnace filters and scheduling driveway resurfacing. Through the years, I have used the services of handymen for precise and heavier jobs. Someone is always available to perform this work!

As with most people I know, my life is many layered...similar to a cake; beginning with a sturdy foundation or base layer of authenticity followed by a multi-skilled and ever-growing resilience middle layer, and topped with an expanding layer of joy and laughter. It has required a lifetime to identify this *is* the life in which I am the happiest and have the highest probability of relaxing and flourishing. With each passing year, I notice I tend to live more self-protectively. These multi-layers combined with the presence of God, Mary, and the Holy Spirit—I value and love my life.

THOUGHTS FOR CONTEMPLATION

1. How do you spend your time after you take care of your medical responsibilities?
2. During an ideal weekend, how would you spend your time and with whom?
3. What are your favorite hobbies?

14

Transitions

This collection of essays is becoming a book. As the transition occurs, the focus of my life has slowly begun to shift. Working with a publishing team has been somewhat complicated since I don't "speak publishing." I have made suggestions to the cover designers which reflect the simplicity of *CANCER HOPE's* thoughts about empowering patients to use their own unique time-tested skills and also to be open to learning new skills as they face their diagnosis and work toward becoming a cancer survivor.

I am thrilled with the book's new cover. I have asked myself, "Is the cover appealing and eye-catching enough to match potential readers' interest?" "How will possible readers respond to the description of the book on the back cover?" Yes, this book is confidence-building when the patient learns he or she already has some of the needed skills to become a successful patient.

A computer-generated copy of the manuscript will be emailed to the publisher today. Yes, I am excited to see the first proof copy (cover and book's interior). It is with excited anticipation that I await the arrival in several weeks.

CANCER HOPE: DISCOVERING SURVI- VOR SKILLS will soon have a life of its own. My thoughts and focus are moving forward from preparation for publication to publication and, finally, to promotion and selling. I am beginning to explore hiring a publicist. I have been reminded as I interview publicists, to review references and also to query them about previous successes and failures within the health genre.

I have remained somewhat cloistered since last summer while in the process of writing and shepherding the book to publication. Developing the book has been a study in both patience and trust in the process. The initial manuscript was without a title until late last fall, just days before the readers received it. I trusted, as I kept rereading the manuscript, that the title would simply pop into my mind. It did. As I reread my oncologist's margin notes, I noticed she kept returning to the word, "hope." Her notes were the key that unlocked the manuscript's title! After the book's title was confirmed, I then saw how well it fit the book. These coincidences continue to contribute to the charm and synchronicity that I love about writing.

As I continue to detach from the sole ownership of *CANCER HOPE*, I am reminded that soon it will become a shared venture with the readers. The book was written with the intention of bringing authenticity, resilience, joy, inspiration, and compassion to the reader. Who will the readers be — patients, their family members, their compassionate friends?

THOUGHTS FOR CONTEMPLATION

1. How do you feel about making voluntary transitions?
2. How do you feel about making involuntary transitions?
3. Who will your supports be as you make transitions?

At the time of the writing of this book, I am gratefully alive and happily engaged in my life. Twelve years ago, I experienced a remarkable evening while saying a final good-bye to my Aunt Bobbie. I brought an informal dinner to the familiar home of my aunt and uncle, Bobbie and Carvel. With the permission of their children, I am sharing this memory of the lovely evening spent with them and two of their three children, Heather and Brandt. Their older son Forrest had returned home earlier in the day.

15

Endings

Twelve years ago, I had the opportunity, quite unexpectedly, to witness and to be an active participant in one of the holiest experience of my life. Word was received from my father that his sister-in-law, Bobbie, was dying. I knew her as a warm, fun-loving, very pretty woman with a ready smile. She and her husband, Carvel, were gracious people who lived in an interesting and artistic home with a natural tree-filled ravine just outside the living room windows. Aunt Bobbie enjoyed wearing the most beautiful one-of-a-kind clothing I have ever seen.

I called my aunt and uncle's home; their daughter, my cousin Heather, answered the phone. She was on leave from her position as a hospital hospice nurse. She had temporarily returned to her parents' home in the suburban neighborhood where she had spent her childhood, to fulfill the mission of providing hospice care to her very sick mother. As we chatted, I offered to bring dinner for their family to their home. Heather accepted my offer and we scheduled dinner for the following evening.

When I arrived the next evening, Heather's brother Brandt who lived with his family in a neighboring suburb, met me and carried the dinner food basket over the driveway bridge to his parents' home. We entered the house and I was greeted by a stunningly touching sight. Aunt Bobbie lay in a raised hospital bed angled to allow her to look out of the living room windows onto the ravine on this cold, moon-lit late January evening. Heather had dressed Aunt Bobbie in a silky pale pink gown and bed jacket. The room was flooded with light from the logs burning in the massive brick fireplace and also from forty or more white candles of every height and shape in the living room and adjoining large dining room.

I approached Aunt Bobbie as the others quietly left the room for the kitchen. I felt grateful that I had this opportunity to share my feelings as I said goodbye to my favorite aunt, a woman of substance and lovely in every way I could imagine.

Joining my two cousins and uncle in the kitchen, we unpacked the food basket, set the table, and assembled dinner. As we enjoyed the Kalamata olives appetizer, we laughed about some of the antiquated kitchen paraphernalia my aunt and uncle had collected and used for many years. Poking around in the fridge, I found Starbucks coffee ice-cream that another cousin, Forrest, had brought earlier in the day before returning to his home. I thought it would be perfect with the chocolate brownies planned for dessert.

As we sat down to our winter chili dinner, Aunt Bobbie was visible just twenty feet away, resting comfortably amidst the candle glow and the sound of the crackling fireplace logs. The four of us reminisced, sharing, and laughing in soft tones. We were brought together unexpectedly by this holy celebration of Bobbie's life. This left me breathless. It was as if God, Mary, and certainly the Holy Spirit had joined in this celebration of life: Bobbie Tefft's life.

As we chatted after dinner, several of her adolescent grandchildren wandered in to speak with her and to say hello to the adults sitting around the dining room table, and then slipped out into the cool night air. I felt privileged and honored to play a small role as I witnessed this holy, holy event. Thanks be to God.

An addendum from cousin Brandt included in his written permission to use "Endings" in *CANCER HOPE*. Brandt offered *his* response to his mother's passing.

"Heather being a hospice nurse knew when mother was about to pass. Thinking it was very soon, she called me and I decided to stay over that night. Heather slept on the couch next to mother in the living room and I was on the floor next to her sleeping on a cushion. During the night there was a knock on the door, so I got up, opened the door and saw three glowing figures. They said they had come for mother. I said sure, she is right here… then I woke up. I stood up and looked at mother, she was still warm. I called to Heather and said to Heather that I think mother had just passed. Heather got up, checked mother, and confirmed that she had just passed."

THOUGHTS FOR CONTEMPLATION

1. What are your feelings after having read this essay?
2. If appropriate, are you comfortable talking with family about "final plans?"
3. If appropriate, is there one specific person with whom you prefer to discuss "final plans?"

16

Resources

MAGAZINES

CONQUER magazine
1249 South River Road, Suite 202
Cranberry NJ 09512
732.992.1891

Coping with Cancer
Published by Media America, Inc
PO Box 682268
Franklin TN 37068.2268
615.791.3859
Email: info@copingmag.com

Cure
PO Box 388
Plainsboro, NJ 08536
800.210.2873

WEBSITES

American Cancer Society
www.cancer.org
800.227.2345

www.choosehope.com
1261 W. Main St
Sun Prairie, WI 53590
888.348.4673

ADULT CANCER TREATMENT CENTERS
Best Hospitals for Cancer
US News Best Hospitals

17

Bibliography

Acquista, Angelo, M.D., and Laurie Anne Vander-molen, *The Mediterranean Prescription Meal Plan and Recipes to Help You Stay Slim and Healthy for the Rest of Your Life*, New York, NY: Ballentine Books, 2006.

Bernhard, Toni, *How to Be Sick A Buddhist-Inspired Guide for the Chronically Ill and Their Caregivers*, Boston, MA: Wisdom Publications, 2010.

Brokaw, Tom, *A Lucky Life Interrupted, A Memoir of Hope*, New York, N.Y: Random House, 2015.

Brooks, David, *The Road to Character*, New York, N.Y: Random House, 2015.

Buchman, Sunny and Paul Buchman, *The Precious Window of Time: Our Journey with Alzheimer's Disease*, Bloomington, IN: AuthorHouse, 2011.

Covey, Stephen, *The Seven Habits of Highly Effective People: Powerful Lessons in Personal Change*, New York, N.Y: Simon and Schuster, 1989.

Didion, Joan, *The Year of Magical Thinking*, New York, N.Y: Alfred Knopf, 2006.

Fennell, Patricia, *The Chronic Illness Workbook Strategies and Solutions for Taking Back Your Life*, *Latham*, *N.Y*: Albany Health Management Publishing, 2012.

Gladwell, Malcolm, *Outliers: The Story of Success*, New York, N.Y: Back Bay Books, 2008.

Housden, Roger, *ten poems to last a lifetime*, HARMONY BOOKS, New York, N.Y: 2004.

Kalanithi, Paul, M.D., *When Breath Becomes Air*, New York, N.Y: Random House, 2016.

Kubler-Ross, Elisabeth, M.D., *Questions and Answers on Death and Dying*, New York, N.Y: Macmillan Publishing, *1974*.

LaMott, Anne, *Help Thanks Wow The Three Essential Prayers*, New York, N.Y: Riverhead. Books, 2012.

LaMott, Anne, *A Handbook of Meaning, Hope, and Repair*, New York, N.Y: Riverhead Books *2013*.

Nhat Hanh, Thich, *Peace Is Every Step The Path of Mindfulness in Everyday Life*, New York, N.Y: Bantam Books, 1991.

Norris, Patricia, Ph.D. and Garrett Porter, *I Choose Life the Dynamics of Visualization and Biofeedback*, Walpole, N.H: Stillpoint Publishing, 1987.

Pausch, Randy, Ph.D., and Jeffrey Maslow, *The Last Lecture*, New York, N.Y: Hyperion, 2008.

Seals, Joy H. and Steven S. Overman, M.D., *You Don't Look Sick Living Well with Invisible Chronic Illness*, New York, N.Y: DemosHEALTH, 2013.

Servan-Schreiber, David, M.D., Ph.D., *Anticancer A New Way of Life*, New York, N.Y: Viking 2010.

Stoddard, Alexandra, *Choosing Happiness Keys to a Joyful Life*, New York, N.Y: Collins, 2002.

Taylor, Jill Bolte, Ph.D., *My Stroke of Insight A Brain Scientist's Personal Journey*, New York, N.Y: Plume Penguin, 2009.

Wilson, Paul, *The Little Book of Calm*, London, England: Penguin Books,1997.

Zeiger, Genie, *How I Find Her a Mother's Dying and a Daughter's Life*, Santa Fe, N.M: Sherman Asher Publishing, 2001.

18

Diane is retired from her small private practice in which she counseled adults with a chemical dependency diagnosis. She has also served her suburban Episcopal church as an Alter Guild member and most recently as a Lay Eucharist Minister. Diane received a B.A. from The Ohio State University and an M.A. in counseling psychology from Antioch University Midwest. While continuing to maintain her Licensed Independent Chemical Dependency Counselor, Clinical Supervisor status (licensed by the State of Ohio), she thoroughly enjoys the freedom and flexibility of being retired. In early retirement, she conceived and then created a colorful hand-knitted fiber arts business, Lainie Alexander Wearable Art. Diane is an almost life-long resident of Upper Arlington, Ohio. Her first memoir, *Humbled by the Gift of Life, Reflections on Receiving a Lung Transplant*, was published in 2012.

19

Acknowledgements

I am baffled and yet not baffled by how friends intuitively knew when to call and when to come to my aid once diagnosed with cancer. Perhaps it was the serious stage 3C endometrial cancer diagnosis or maybe it was the memory of an earlier loss of a beloved family member or friend that motivated them. Most likely, these friends are quite simply kind and compassionate people who listen to their hearts.

My chemo infusions always began as early in the morning as possible. By eight o'clock on most chemo mornings, I was the passenger in a cheerful friend's car on the way to the Bing Center's outpatient chemo drop-off. A grateful thank you to those early-rising friends, who were transporters extraordinaire: Lou Ann, Julie, Lois, Joyce, and Gretchen. Because I am so needle-phobic, the drivers almost always had to nudge me to exit their cars so I could pass through the Bing Cancer Center entrance as I headed for the third floor infusion area.

Seasoned garden designer, Diane, knew exactly how to be helpful *and* have fun. Diane was assisted by both her gardening crew and trusted gardener-friend Susie. The newly planted garden rapidly grew into a blooming profusion of colorful perennial flowers bordering the walkway from the driveway to my olive green front door. Flowers and colorful twisting vines are always blooming and appear so welcoming against the khaki color of the exterior wood siding and the large centered stone fireplace.

I had the extraordinary good fortune to have a cancer mentor. She preceded me by several years as being diagnosed with stage 3C endometrial cancer and also becoming a cancer survivor.

While her treatment occurred at another local cancer-designated hospital, our experiences mirrored each others. Whenever I felt exhausted or overwhelmed, I would think of her, and her enviable creative ability to be herself and at the same time see the humor in life's health and other challenges. My uncomfortable feelings would evaporate and a sense of calm would take over. She remains a kind role model who has consistently made it possible to "see" hope.

Once the manuscript was finished late last fall, it was time to ask two well-read friends to be "readers." Although the manuscript was initially edited by Gretchen off and on as I was still writing the essays, the readers' goal was to review the individual essays and then see how they fitted together as a unified refined read. Once the readers were finished, they asked provocative questions: "Do you need to write so much about your transplant in this cancer-themed story?" and "Why is authenticity so important and why is it a part of the story?" Both readers

(Lynn and Susannah) were fortunately also able to catch grammatical and spelling errors that had slipped through the hands of others. For Lynn and Susannah, reading the manuscript was gratefully squeezed into pre-holiday activities. Thank you, Thank you.

I asked for and was given a most generous gift, when I inquired if my oncologist would be willing to read the manuscript. How this busy physician was able to introduce this concentrated activity into her life during end-of-the-year holiday and family activities, I will never know. I do feel grateful for her time, support, and oncology skills. Her side bar or margin comments were, at times, humorous and always valuable.

I felt the steady presence and support of my spiritual director Susannah as we spoke every three or four weeks. I *always* felt she was floating somewhere in the background of my life. She has an enviable sense of humor and she is also an expert listener, hearing what is being said as well as what hasn't been said.

Son Andrew and his children were consistently in the background of my life. They assumed responsibility for all the needed tree and bush trimming and removal of the endless unwanted weeds that kept reappearing despite the dark mulch ground cover. I always looked forward to my grandchildren's presence and clearly appreciated their gardening and other home maintenance skills. My sister Melissa and cousin Heather remained in touch through update phone calls filled with positive thoughts and healing prayers.

A gift of a different sort appeared unexpectedly when Gretchen introduced me to the world of writers. It was Gretchen who extended an invitation to join the first writing critique group as well as the second group whose focus was on writing lovely essays for publication. I wasn't aware of how little I knew until I was exposed to these experienced polished and published writers who *sold* their essays. *Wow!* I was overwhelmed by their perceptive critique comments.

Thank you, for this introduction into a fascinating new world.

Blessings upon Christie for her timely appearance and precision-driven editing talents.

Finally, to the staff of Ohio Health's Riverside Methodist Hospital's Bing Cancer Center...a certified member of MD Anderson Cancer Network, thank you for your consistently well-trained, compassionate, and superior staff. In addition to chemo infusions and radiation, I also benefitted from the integrative medicine services (massage and acupuncture) and Over My Head Boutique where patients find wigs, head coverings, and mastectomy wear. My family and I send a deeply felt Thank You to all the Bing Cancer Center staff.

20

Photographs

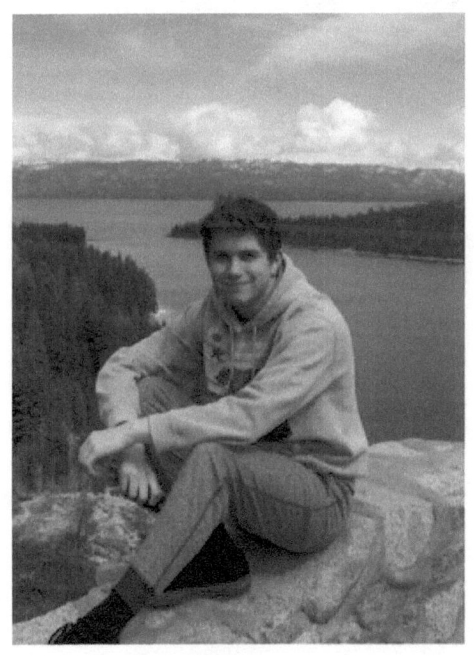

ALEX

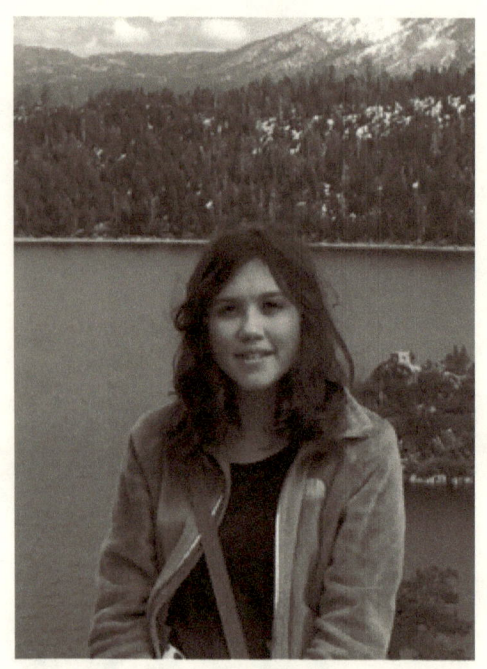

KATIE

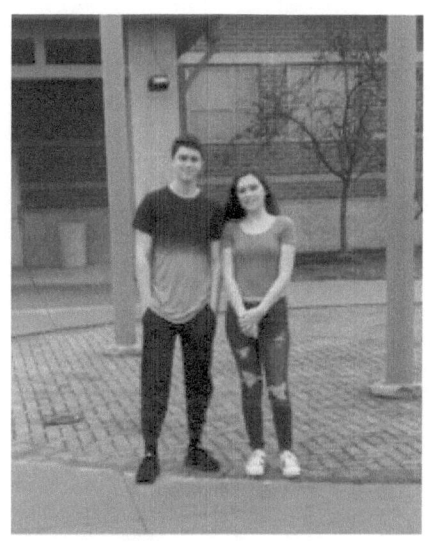

ALEX AND KATIE

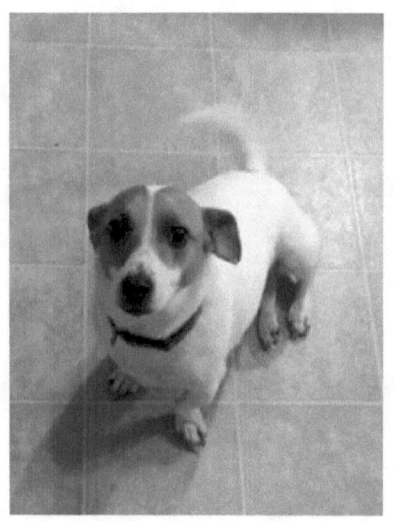

EDDIE

www.ingramcontent.com/pod-product-compliance
Lightning Source LLC
Chambersburg PA
CBHW050450290526
45786CB00006B/2228